SOMATIC EXERCISES FOR WEIGHT LOSS

UNLOCKING THE POTENTIAL OF BODY AWARENESS FOR A SLIMMER - HEALTHIER YOU.

MARY S. JAHN

Contents

Introduction to Somatics

- **Understanding Somatics**
- **The Mind-Body Connection**
- **Benefits of Somatic Exercises**
- **Preparing for Your Somatic Journey**

Foundational Movements

- **breathing techniques**
- **Core Engagement**
- **Grounding Exercises**
- **Dynamic Stretching**

Somatics for Upper Body

- **Shoulder Rolls**
- **Arm Swings**

- **Tai Chi and Qigong**
- **Walking Meditation**
- **Progressive Muscle Relaxation (PMR)**

Integrating Somatics into Daily Life

- **Mindful Morning Start**
- **Conscious Commuting**
- **Desk Dynamics**
- **Evening Unwind**
- **Somatic Breaks**

Somatic exercises for emotional balance

- **Grounding**
- **Diaphragmatic Breathing**
- **Pendulation**
- **Palming**
- **Self-Hug**
- **Mindful Walking**
- **Body Scan**
- **Progressive Muscle Relaxation**
- **Visualization**
- **Cathartic Movement**

Somatic Exercise for Weight Loss

- **Grounding**
- **Diaphragmatic Breathing**
- **Pelvic Tilts**

- **<u>Self-Hug</u>**
- **<u>Somatic Walking</u>**
- **<u>Somatic Squats</u>**
- **<u>Arm Swings</u>**
- **<u>Cat-Cow Stretch</u>**
- **<u>Grounding Exercises</u>**
- **<u>Breathwork</u>**
- **<u>Posture Exercises</u>**
- **<u>Somatic Experiencing</u>**
- **<u>Eye Movement Desensitization and Reprocessing (EMDR)</u>**
- **<u>EXTRA 1-month workouts plan</u>**

<u>Conclusion</u>

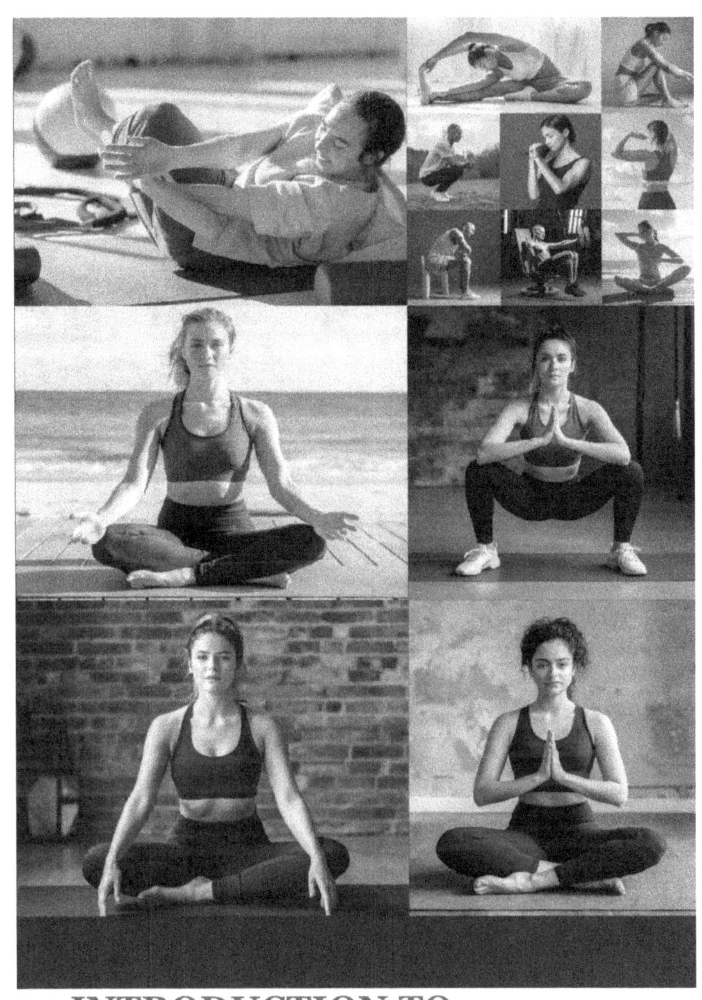

INTRODUCTION TO SOMATICS

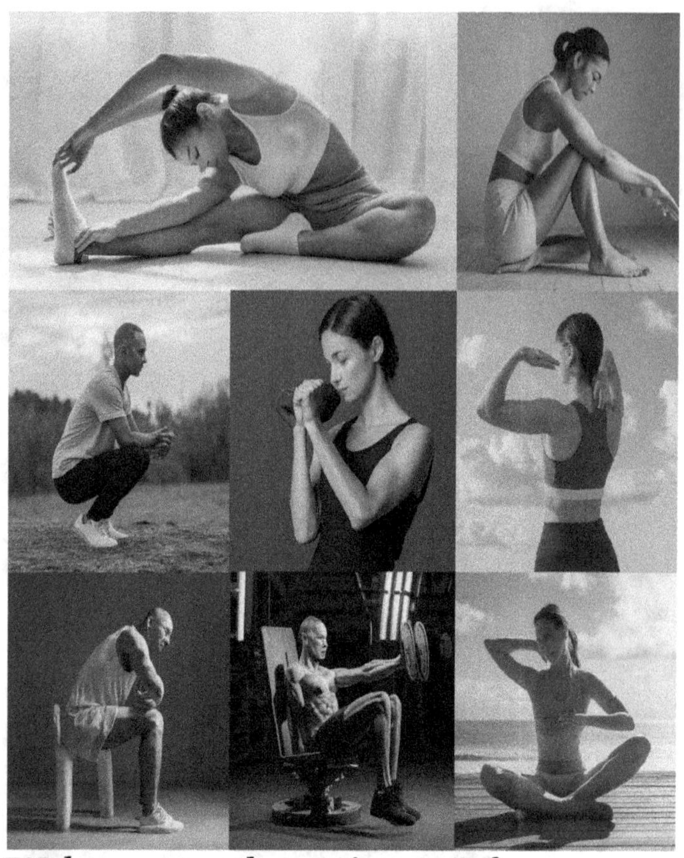

Welcome to the universe of Somatics, a groundbreaking practice where the excursion of weight reduction rises above the physical and turns into an amicable dance between brain and body. Somatics, derived from the Greek word 'soma' signifying 'the living body,' isn't simply an activity routine; it's a way of thinking, a method of correcting the body to move uninhibitedly and proficiently.

In a general public overflowing with handy solutions and moment results, Somatics stands apart as a guide of mindfulness and delicate advancement. It welcomes you to dial back, to listen eagerly to the murmurs of your body, and to answer with developments that are essentially as normal as a much-needed refresher in the first part of the daylight.

As you leave on this way, you'll find practices that don't simply intend to consume calories but to stir the faculties. These developments are intended to deliver strain, improve portability, and develop an underpinning of center fortitude that upholds your actual objectives as well as your profound prosperity.

Through the pages of this book, you'll figure out how to develop a relationship with your body that is established in graciousness and regard. You'll track down happiness in the straightforwardness of a stretch, the beauty of a stance, and the force of a muscle participating in calm strength. This is the substance of Somatics - a training that doesn't yell its triumphs but rather, celebrates them in the quiet certainty of a body in balance.

Thus, take a full breath, and we should start this excursion together. An excursion where each step is a demonstration of confidence, every development a sonnet, and the location a spot where your body and heart coincide in gorgeous, weightless concordance.

I trust this presentation reverberates with the soul of your book and gives a warm and welcoming section into the extraordinary universe of Somatics works out.

UNDERSTANDING SOMATICS

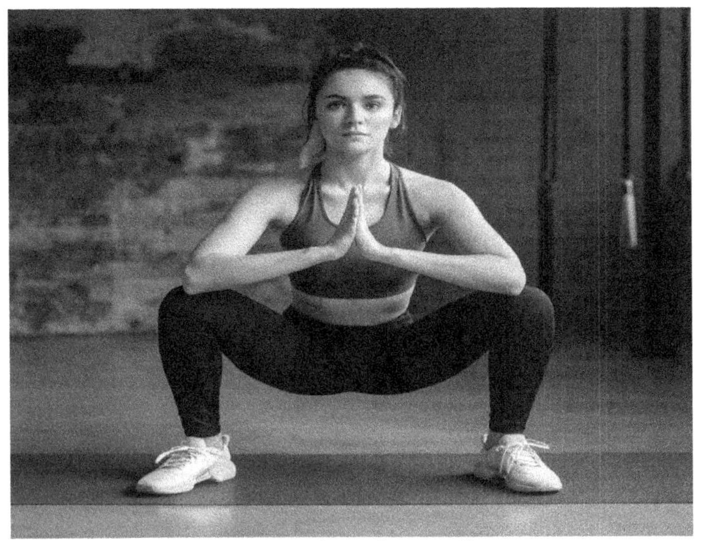

Leave on an excursion into the core of development with Somatics works out, where each movement is a private discussion with your body. Somatics, a term that praises the no-nonsense element that is our body, isn't just about the workout; it's about association, mindfulness, and the sensitive dance between psyche and muscle.

The Embodiment of Somatics practices is the verse of actual structure, the delicate touch that stirs torpid muscles, and the delicate murmur that quiets the overactive psyche. They are developments as well as articulations of taking care of oneself that reverberate through the passageways of our being, welcoming us to move with expectation and effortlessness.

The Act of Presence In the act of Somatics, presence is fundamental. It's tied in with being completely at the time, with every breath and each stretch. It's tied in with respecting the body's insight, permitting it to direct us through developments that mend, balance, and revive. This is where the human articulation in Somatics sparkles — through the careful consideration we provide for all aspects of ourselves.

The Ensemble of Development Envision your body as an orchestra, with each muscle a performer prepared to have its impact. Somatic practices are the guide's rod, coordinating an agreeable execution that reverberates with the song of prosperity. It's an orchestra where each note matters, and the music is the liquid language of well-being and imperativeness.

The Groundbreaking Power Somatics is extraordinary, not because it changes what our identity is, but because it uncovers the full range of our true capacity. It helps us to shed the layers of strain and limitation, to stand tall in the radiance of our actual stance, and to move with the opportunity that comes from the inside.

The Human Touch As you dive into Somatics works out, recollect that they are a gift you give yourself — a demonstration of the conviction that your body has the right to move effortlessly. According to a human touch, "I'm here, I am mindful, and I'm prepared to embrace the magnificence of development in its most perfect structure."

This prologue to Somatics practices is made to give a profound comprehension of the work, underscoring the human association with our actual structure and the careful way to deal with the development that characterizes Somatics. May it move and guide perusers to a more adjusted and merciful relationship with their bodies.

THE MIND-BODY CONNECTION

In the woven artwork of well-being and health, the brain-body association is the brilliant string that winds around together the physical and the mental, the unmistakable and the elusive. It is significant to figure out that our considerations, sentiments, and convictions essentially affect our natural working, and that our physical encounters, thus, impact our psychological state.

The Dance of Exchange Envision the psyche and body in a never-ending dance, every development a discourse between the two. The psyche murmurs an idea, and the body answers with a sensation. The body encounters a touch, and the psyche interprets it into feeling. This dance is the quintessence of the psyche-body association — a delightful, perplexing interaction that shapes our experience of life.

The Force of Discernment Our insights form our existence. How we decipher pressure, delight, or torment isn't simply a psychological activity; it shows genuinely in our bodies. An uplifting perspective can support our safe framework, while constant pressure can wear it out. This association advises us that sustaining our psychological nursery is pretty much as critical as focusing on our actual vessel.

The Agreement of Wellbeing isn't simply the shortfall of illness; it's the concordance of the psyche and body. The tranquil snapshots of care quite a hustling heart, the full breaths that move a strained back, and the chuckling that eases up a weighty soul. As one lies the key to a day-to-day existence lived completely and a body loved profoundly.

The Human Touch As you investigate the psyche-body association through Somatics, make sure to carry a human touch to your training. Be caring to yourself, patient with your advancement, and merciful towards your body's signs. Commend the little triumphs, the unpretentious changes in mindfulness, and the delicate arrival of strain. These are the human articulations of a profound and significant association with oneself.

This segment plans to give perusers a rich comprehension of the psyche-body association, underlining the human part of our cooperation with our actual selves. May it act as a motivation for a more careful and associated way to deal with well-being and health.

BENEFITS OF SOMATIC EXERCISES

Substantial activities offer an abundance of advantages that upgrade both the physical and mental parts of well-being. Here is an extensive glance at the advantages of integrating Substantial activities into your daily schedule:

ACTUAL ADVANTAGES

Further developed Adaptability: Normal practice can prompt more noteworthy simplicity and scope of movement in the joints.

Upgraded Stance: By zeroing in on the body's inward sensations, Physical activities can assist with revising poor postural habits.

Expanded Development Quality: These activities empower more productive and effortless developments, diminishing the gamble of injury.

Muscle Unwinding: Somatics help the body to deliver pressure and snugness, prompting a looser state.

MENTAL AND PROFOUND ADVANTAGES

Stress Decrease: The careful idea of Physical activities assists lower with pushing levels and advances a feeling of well-being2.

Better Rest and Unwinding: Taking part in these activities

can further develop rest quality and help in relaxation.

Upgraded Psyche Body Association: Somatics cultivate a more profound consciousness of the body, which can prompt a more agreeable brain-body relationship.

Profound Delivery: The training can work with the arrival of repressed feelings, adding to home balance.

IN GENERAL PROSPERITY

Help with discomfort: By retraining the sensory system, Substantial activities can mitigate persistent agony and discomfort2.

Further developed Equilibrium: These activities can help keep up with and further develop balance, which is vital for all age groups.

More noteworthy Body Mindfulness: Members frequently experience an expanded comprehension of their body's necessities and capabilities.

Integrating Substantial activities into your day-to-day existence can prompt extraordinary outcomes, genuinely as well as in your general way of dealing with well-being and health. They welcome you to investigate development with interest and sympathy, prompting a more adjusted and satisfying relationship with your body.

PREPARING FOR YOUR SOMATIC JOURNEY

It's like setting sail on a calm sea on your Somatic journey, where the waves of movement take you to a place of balance and well-being. You can get ready for this journey that will change you:

Creating a Conducive Environment Choose an environment that is peaceful, inviting, and free of distractions. Your haven, a place where the conversation between your mind and body takes center stage and the outside world fades away.

Gathering Your Tools While somatic exercises don't require any special equipment, you might want to bring a yoga mat or a soft surface to lie on, comfortable clothes that let you move freely, and maybe a blanket to keep you warm when you relax.

Setting Goals Approach your practice with a goal in mind. Think about what you want to accomplish, whether it's less stress, less pain, or just a moment of peace. You will be guided by this intention, which will keep you focused on your goal.

EMBRACING PATIENCE YOUR COMPANION

on this journey is patience. In somatics, awareness and movement are developed gradually rather than in a flash. Maintain self-patience as you develop and learn. Pay attention to the subtle cues your body gives you by listening to it.

It communicates through sensations and levels of comfort, directing you toward movements that best serve you. You will acquire the soma language by listening.

Consistency is essential when practicing regularly. Even if it only takes a few minutes, schedule Somatic exercises into your daily routine. The benefits will grow and the mind-body connection will get stronger with practice. Looking for Direction If you're new to Somatics, consider looking for direction from a certified teacher who can acquaint you with the activities and guarantee you're performing them securely and successfully.

Last but not least, accept the journey with an open heart. Celebrate each step forward, each breath, and each movement. You are about to join a dance of life, not just a journey of the body but also of the soul. yeah

You are now prepared to begin your Somatic journey with these preparations in place. May it be a path of joyous movement, healing, and discovery.

FOUNDATIONAL MOVEMENTS

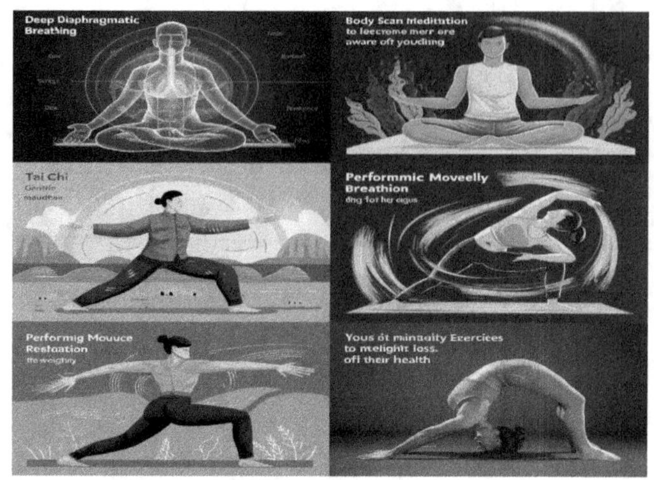

Breathing techniques

The goal is to improve body oxygenation and reduce stress.

How to Do It: Relax and lie down. Place one hand on your abdomen and one on your chest. Inhale profoundly through your nose, permitting your mid-region to ascend higher than your chest. Through the mouth, slowly exhale. Reduces heart rate, promotes full oxygen exchange, and has the potential to lower blood pressure.

Core Engagement

Identifying areas of tension and encouraging relaxation is the goal.

How to Do It: Find a quiet spot where you can

comfortably sit or lie down. Shut your eyes and intellectually filter your body from head to toe. Breathe into any areas of tension you notice, allowing them to relax. Increases body awareness and can help identify and release muscle tension caused by stress.

Grounding Exercises

The goal is to promote deep relaxation and muscle relaxation.

How to do: Tense eatch muscle bunch for 5 seconds and afterward discharge. Work your way up to the head from the toes.

Benefits: Assists in lessening focusing on uneasiness, further develops rest quality, and can support torment management.

Careful Strolling: The goal is to strengthen the mind-body connection by connecting movement and mindfulness. Method: Walk at your own pace. Center around the impression of your feet contacting the ground.

When your mind wanders, gently bring it back to the sensation of walking. Align your breathing with your steps. Cardiovascular health, stress reduction, and improved focus and concentration are some of the advantages.

Dynamic Stretching

Reason: To deliver close-to-home pressure through active work.

How to Do It: Don't judge yourself and let your body move freely. Dance, shake, or move in any capacity that feels regular, relinquishing put away feelings.

Emotional release, increased energy, and a sense of lightness and freedom are some of the benefits. Not only are these fundamental movements helpful for losing weight, but they also help you develop a deeper connection with your body.

They advocate taking a holistic approach to health, emphasizing self-care for both physical and emotional well-being. A more balanced and satisfying life can result from incorporating these practices into your daily routine.

SOMATICS FOR UPPER BODY

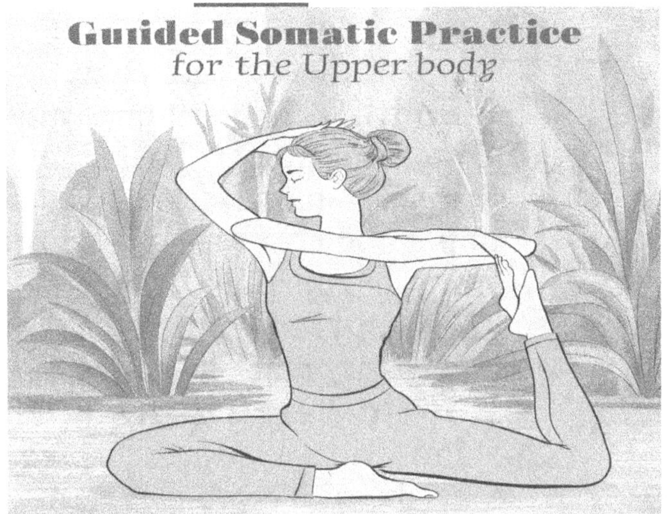

Shoulder Rolls

The goal is to let go of tension in the neck and shoulders.

Method: Stand or sit comfortably. Gradually roll your shoulders forward, up, and afterward back in a round movement. After performing this several times, turn around. Improves shoulder mobility and may help ease stiffness in the neck1.

Arm Swings

The goal is to work the upper back and arm muscles.

Instructions: Stand with your feet shoulder-width apart. Swing your arms across your body, one over the other, and then back out to the sides. Extend your arms to the sides. Keep moving rhythmically.

Benefits: Helps tone the arms and upper back1 and increases blood flow to the upper body.

Chest Expander

The goal is to open the chest and make breathing easier.

How to Perform It: Sit or stand with a straight spine. Straighten your arms, interlace your fingers behind your back, and gently lift your arms while expanding your chest outward and upward.

Benefits: Supports further breathing and stretches the chest muscles.

Neck Stretch

The goal is to relax the neck and upper shoulders.

How to Perform It: Sit straight and comfortably. Bring your ear toward your shoulder and gently tilt your head to one side. After holding for a few seconds, switch sides. Reduces neck tension and may assist in preventing headaches[1].

Upper Back Release

Reason: To calm and stretch the upper back. The most effective method to Make it happen is to sit on the floor with your legs crossed. Walk forward with your hands on the floor in front of you and let your chest sink toward the ground.

Benefits: Promotes relaxation and stretches the upper back and shoulder blades[1].

These gentle but effective exercises focus on releasing tension and strengthening the upper body, both of which can help you lose weight and speed up your metabolism. Keep in mind to pay attention to your body and exercise within your range of motion.

SOMATICS FOR CORE STRENGTH

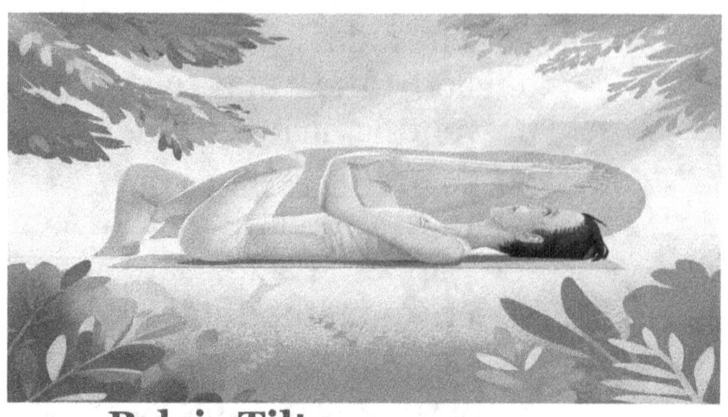

- **Pelvic Tilts**

The goal is to strengthen and engage the deep core muscles.

How to Perform It: Lie on your back with your feet flat on the ground and your knees bent. Flatten your lower back against the floor after gently arching it. Concentrating on the sensation in your pelvic area, slowly repeat this movement. Improves stability in the lower back and strengthens the abdominal muscles.

The Cat-Cow Stretch

To improve core awareness and spinal flexibility.

How to do: Begin your hands and knees in a tabletop position. As you inhale, raise your head and tailbone while arching your back down (like a cow). As you tuck your chin into your chest and round your back (cat), exhale.

Benefits: Strengthens the core muscles and encourages movement of the spine1.

Supine Leg Extensions

The objective is to test the core muscles' stability. The most effective method to

Make it happen: Lie on your back with your knees twisted. While keeping your lower back pressed to the floor, slowly extend one leg at a time. Concentrate on the movement's control and sensation. Boosts leg strength and improves core engagement.

Seated Twists

Reason: To work on rotational versatility and center strength. Instructions to Make it happen: Sit tall with your legs crossed. Position one hand behind you and the other on the knee in front of you. As you look over your shoulder, gently twist your torso. After holding for a few seconds, switch sides. Increases spinal rotation and muscle strength in the oblique region.

<u>**Bridge Pose**</u>

The goal is to open the hip flexors while strengthening the glutes and core. How to Perform It: Lie on your back with your feet hip-width apart and your knees bent. As you lift your hips toward the ceiling, press your feet onto the floor. If you need support, put your hands under your back.

Benefits: Develops center and lower body fortitude, and can lighten pressure in the hips. The ability to be mindful and focused on the internal experience of movement is essential to the success of these somatic exercises for core strength and weight loss. Make sure to play out these activities with consideration regarding structure and the sensations in your body.

SOMATICS FOR LOWER BODY

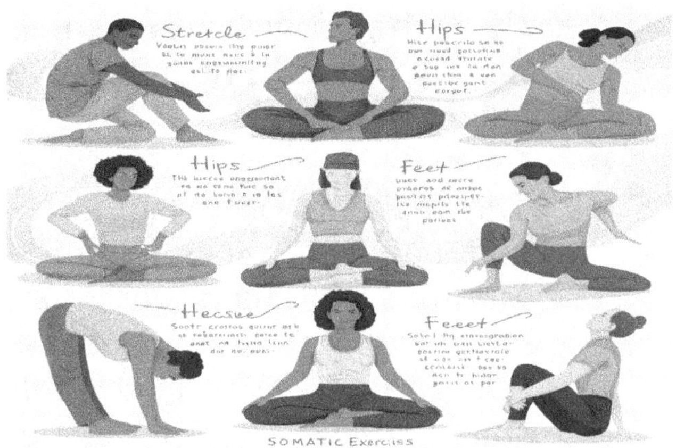

Circular Hips

The objective is to lessen tension and improve hip mobility.

Step 1: Stand with your feet shoulder-width apart. Place your hands on your hips and slowly make a clockwise and then a counterclockwise circle around your hips. Maintain control and smoothness in the movement. Improves hip joint flexibility and may help alleviate lower back pain.

Leg Lifts: The goal is to stabilize the hips and strengthen the thigh muscles.

How to Perform It: Lie on your side with straight legs. Lower the top leg back down after lifting it straight. Before switching sides, repeat several times.

Benefits: Tones the thigh muscles and can help improve balance.

Foot Rolls

The goal is to prevent injuries and enhance ankle mobility. Method: Stand or sit comfortably. Take one foot off the ground and slowly roll your ankle in a circle. Complete a few turns in the two bearings before changing to the next lower leg.

Benefits: Improves ankle flexibility and **circulation.**

To Get Up Squat

The goal is to work the major lower body muscle groups.Instructions: Stand with your feet shoulder-width apart. Push through your heels to get back to standing after lowering yourself into a squat with your knees bent.

Benefits: Strengthens the core, legs, and glutes, which may help you lose weight1. Raises of the Calves: The objective is to enhance stability in the lower leg and strengthen the calf muscles.

Step 1: Stand with your feet shoulder-width apart. Ascend onto the wads of your feet, lifting your impact points as high as could be expected. Lower down with control.

Benefits: Helps stabilize the ankles and tones the calves1. The key to the effectiveness of these Somatic exercises in reducing weight and enhancing body awareness is their focus on the internal experience of movement. Make sure to play out these activities with consideration regarding structure and the sensations in your body.

<u>**Somatic Flow Routines**</u>

The following are five Somatic Flow Routines that can help you lose weight:

<u>**Gentle Flow to Wake Up**</u>

The objective is to gently arouse the mind and body in preparation for the following day.

How to Do It: Begin by lightly stretching in bed and breathing deeply through the diaphragm. Move on to standing stretches that work your entire body. Benefits: Increments flow, supports energy levels, and improves mental lucidity.

Late morning Re-energize Stream

The goal is to re-energize the body and let go of tension from the morning.

How to Do It: Start with dynamic movements like swinging your arms and twisting your torso, then go for a short walk or do some light aerobics. It aids in overcoming the midday slump, enhances focus, and maintains metabolic rate, among other advantages.

Evening Relaxation Flow

After the activities of the day, the goal is to move the body into a state of relaxation.

The most effective method to Make it happen: Take part in a progression of slow, smooth motions, for example, Kendo or delicate yoga presents, zeroing in on the breath and delivering muscle pressure. It helps digestion, promotes relaxation, and prepares the body for a restful night's sleep.

Flow of Stress-Release

The goal is to reduce stress and the physical symptoms it causes.

How to Do It: To get rid of stress from your body, use techniques like progressive muscle relaxation, visualization, and mindful meditation. Boosts weight loss efforts, lowers cortisol levels and reduces emotional eating.

Flow of Dynamic Movement

The objective is to encourage weight loss and enhance physical fitness.

How to do: Consolidate components of dance, combative techniques, and plyometric activities to make a dynamic and fun daily practice.

Benefits: Consumes calories, works on cardiovascular wellbeing, and upgrades body mindfulness.

These routines not only help people lose weight but also improve their overall health. They enable you to connect with your body and recognize its needs, which leads to a healthier lifestyle, and they encourage a mindful approach to movement.

Advanced Methods of the Body Due to their emphasis on internal awareness and stress reduction, advanced somatic techniques for weight loss can be particularly effective. These techniques involve a deeper level of mind-body integration.

ADVANCED SOMATIC TECHNIQUES

Physical Yoga

The goal is to combine the body awareness of Somatics with the mindfulness of yoga.

How to Do It: Instead of striving for perfect form, focus on the internal experience of the movement while performing traditional yoga poses. Improves metabolic function, reduces stress, and increases flexibility.

Dance and Development Treatment (DMT):

The goal is to use dance as a way to express and let go of emotions.

How to Do It: Move to music without choreography

and in a way that reflects your feelings.

Benefits: Energizes close-to-home delivery, which can diminish pressure-related eating and weight gain.

Qigong and Tai Chi

Reason: To advance energy stream and equilibrium inside the body.

How to Do It: Focus on breath control and slow, deliberate movements when practicing these martial arts. Improves balance and muscle tone, as well as the possibility of lowering body fat.

Strolling Reflection

The goal is to combine the mental clarity of meditation with the physical benefits of walking.

How to Do It: Walk slowly and carefully, paying attention to how each step feels and how your breath feels. Improves cardiovascular health, reduces stress, and supports weight loss efforts.

PMR, or progressive muscle relaxation

Reason: To let strain out of the muscles deliberately. How to Perform It: Tend each muscle group for a few seconds, then move through the entire body to release the tension.

Physical stress can be reduced, and stress-related overeating can be prevented.

These high-level strategies not only help weight reduction by further developing body mindfulness and diminishing pressure yet in addition add to generally speaking prosperity and a more agreeable relationship with the body.

INTEGRATING SOMATICS INTO DAILY LIFE

Somatic practices can be incorporated into your routine in the following five ways.

- **Mindful Start to the Day**

With an emphasis on body awareness, the goal is to set a positive mood for the day.

How to Do It: Start your day by breathing through your diaphragm or gently stretching while you are still in bed. Take note of how your body moves and feels. The benefits include less stiffness in the morning, increased circulation, and mental and physical preparation for the day ahead.

- **Conscious Travel**

The goal is to take advantage of the time spent traveling to practice mindfulness and reduce stress.

How to Do It: If you're a passenger, do body scanning and deep breathing exercises. Focus on the sensation of your feet touching the ground when you are walking. Benefits: Improves decision-making, including food choices, by reducing stress and increasing mental clarity.

- **Work area Elements**

To prevent the negative effects of sitting for an extended period and to maintain metabolic activity.

How to Do It: Perform seated somatic exercises like neck rolls, shoulder shrugs, and wrist stretches every hour. Benefits: Keeps muscles drawn in, further develops pose, and can forestall the drowsiness related to sitting excessively long.

- **Evening Relax**

Reason: To deliver the day's strain and change into a serene night. The most effective method to Make it happen is to participate in a Physical stream normal or some Kendo developments to loosen up both the psyche and body. Relaxation, support for digestion, and preparation for a restful night's sleep are all advantages.

- **Physical Breaks**

The goal is to incorporate brief, frequent Somatic exercises throughout the day to maintain engagement between the mind and body.

How to Do It: Set reminders so that you remember to take brief breaks for breathing or mindful movement exercises.

Benefits: Keeps a steady degree of active work, which is key for weight reduction, and keeps the psyche-body association dynamic for the day.

You can achieve weight loss and a healthier lifestyle on a

long-term and enjoyable path by incorporating Somatic exercises into your daily routine.

These practices assist in dealing with weighting as well as working on general prosperity by cultivating a more profound association with your body and its necessities.

Exercises for the body's emotional well-being Somatic exercises are a type of therapy that involves the mind and body and focuses on physical movements to help relieve stress and restore emotional equilibrium.

SOMATIC EXERCISES FOR EMOTIONAL BALANCE

Ten detailed explanations of somatic exercises are as follows:

1. Grounding: The motivation behind establishing is to reconnect with your body and the current second. Take a few deep breaths, stand or sit comfortably, and feel your feet on the ground to accomplish this. Stability and calmness are among the advantages.

Diaphragmatic Breathing: This exercise aims to promote relaxation while reducing stress. Place one hand on your belly and one on your chest while lying down or sitting comfortably. Exhale slowly after inhaling deeply and expanding your belly like a balloon. Anxiety is reduced and focus is improved as a result.

Pendulation: The objective here is to see the body's regular mood. Move your attention away from a body sensation, such as tightness, and then back to it, like a pendulum. Recognizing and releasing physical tension is made easier by this.

Palming: To rest and reset your eyes, rub your palms together until they're warm, and afterward delicately place them over your shut eyes. The darkness and warmth can calm the nervous system.

Self-Hug: Gently squeeze yourself while wrapping your arms around yourself.

Oxytocin, a hormone that boosts feelings of well-being, may be released as a result, mimicking the comfort of being embraced.

Mindful walking: involves moving slowly and deliberately while paying attention to how each step feels. This can assist with establishing you in the present and diminish sensations of overpowering.

Body Scan: Focus on each part of your body, starting at the top of your head and working your way down to your toes. This can help you find areas of tension and help you relax in general.

Progressive Muscle Relaxation: Start with your toes and work your way up to your head, tense, and then relax each muscle group in your body. This can improve the quality of your sleep and reduce physical stress.

Perception: Envision a serene scene or a protected spot. Focus on this mental image with every sense you have. This can help you focus on something else and help you feel more peaceful.

Cathartic Movement: Let your body move freely and without thinking about it, releasing any tension. This can assist in the release of bottled-up emotions and boost energy levels.

These exercises are meant to help you become more aware of the sensations in your body and use that awareness to let go of tension in your body and mind. An increased sense of calm and emotional control can result from consistent practice.

Keep in mind that the most important thing to do when doing somatic exercises is to approach them with curiosity and without judging, allowing your body to lead you toward healing and balance.

SOMATIC EXERCISE FOR WEIGHT LOSS

Grounding: This includes deliberately fixing and afterward leisurely delivering muscles, which can assist in lessening muscling strain and further developing adaptability, supporting weight reduction by advancing more productive development patterns. Deep abdominal breathing encourages full oxygen exchange and can help reduce stress, which is frequently linked to weight gain.

Diaphragmatic Breathing: Connecting with the center muscles through pelvic slants can further develop stance and center strength, adding to more readily body arrangement and weight management.

Pendulation: By lying on your back and gently stretching your hamstrings, you can loosen up the tightness in your back and legs, which may help you avoid overeating because you're stressed or uncomfortable.

Pelvic Tilts: Focusing on the sensation of each step while walking can help you lose weight and become more mindful.

Self-Hug: Building strength and burning calories can both be aided by performing squats mindfully and paying attention to the movement and sensation of the muscles.

Somatic Walking: This exercise involves gently swinging the arms. It has the potential to help loosen the shoulder girdle and alleviate the tension in the upper body that can be linked to emotional eating.

Somatic Squats: In a cat-cow stretch, you alternate between arching and rounding your back. This can help you manage stress and lose weight by making your spine more flexible and reducing tension.

Arm Swings: Gentle twisting can aid in detoxification and digestion, both of which are helpful for weight loss.

Cat-Cow Stretch: Focusing on relaxation while lying on your back with your knees bent and feet flat on the ground can support weight loss goals by reducing stress and tension throughout.

Grounding Exercises: The goal of these exercises is to make a strong connection to the ground, which can help with balance and stability. Establishing can likewise decrease pressure, which is frequently connected to weight gain.

Breathwork: Controlled breathing exercises can help you lose weight by increasing oxygen flow, increasing energy, and reducing stress.

Posture Exercises: These exercises have the potential to improve breathing and digestion, both of which are essential for successful weight management.

Somatic Experiencing: This type of treatment includes the delicate arrival of actual pressure and injury put away in the body, which can prompt superior close-to-home prosperity and back weight reduction efforts. The motivation behind these activities is to cultivate a more profound association between the brain and the body, prompting an uplifted feeling of mindfulness and control.

<u>Eye Movement Desensitization and Reprocessing (EMDR):</u> Albeit fundamentally a mental treatment, EMDR can help in handling and delivering profound pressure, which might add to weight reduction by lessening pressure-related eating behaviors. By strengthening the connection between the mind and body and by reducing stress, these exercises not only contribute to a healthier weight but also improve overall well-being. Integrating these practices into your daily routine can be a useful component of a comprehensive weight loss strategy.

<u>EXTRA WEIGHT LOSS-SUPPORTING SOMATIC WORKOUT PLAN FOR ONE MONTH</u>

To assist you in your journey toward a healthier body and mind, this plan emphasizes stress reduction and mindful movement.

Week 1 An Overview of Somatics Monday: 20-minute Body Scan Meditation Yoga Flow for 30 minutes on Tuesday Rest or 20-minute mindful walking on Wednesday Thursday: PMR (progressional muscle relaxation) Friday: Essential Pilates Mat Activities (30 minutes) Saturday: Jujitsu Nuts and bolts (30 minutes) Sunday: Relax and think

Week 2 Making People More Aware Routine for somatic stretching on Monday Tuesday: Balance-Building Hatha Yoga Wednesday: Rest or Nature Walk (30 minutes) PMR and visualization on Thursday (30 minutes) Friday: Pilates with Spotlight on Center (30 minutes) Dance and Movement Therapy on Saturday (30 minutes) Sunday: Relax and think

Week 3 Strengthening the Relationship Monday: Breathwork-based advanced body scan Vinyasa Yoga Flow on Tuesday (30 minutes)

Wednesday: Rest or Comfortable Swim (30 minutes) Thursday: Physical Development Investigation (30 minutes) Friday: Pilates with Balls and Bands as props Aikido or fundamentals of martial arts on Saturday Sunday: Relax and think

Week 4 Combination and Practice Monday: 45-minute full-body somatics routine Tuesday: Power Yoga Meeting (30 minutes) Rest or active recovery (Yin Yoga) on Wednesday Thursday: Somatics paired with cognitive exercises Friday: 45-minute Advanced Pilates Sequence Saturday: 45-minute ecstatic dance session Sunday: Take a Break, Think, and Make Plans A 5-minute warm-up and 5-minute cool-down should be part of each session.

Keep hydrated and pay attention to your body, adjusting the intensity as necessary. For best results, this workout plan must be combined with a healthy diet and enough sleep. Consider consulting a somatic exercise specialist for a more individualized plan or to meet specific needs. Enjoy your journey toward a healthier and more connected you!

CONCLUSION

Let's take a moment to reflect on the journey we've taken together as we close out this journey through "The Complete Somatic Exercises for Weight Loss." This book was more than just a collection of exercises; it was a call to dance with your own body, a dance of discovery, awareness, and transformation.

Embracing the Somatic Way You've learned to listen to your muscles' whispers and your breath's rhythm, discovering in them the harmony of health and movement. Every section was a bit nearer to understanding that weight reduction isn't a fight but an equilibrium — an equilibrium of supporting the body, quieting the psyche, and feeding the spirit.

The Excursion Go on As you close this book, recall that your physical excursion doesn't end here. It continues with each conscious step you take, each conscious breath you take, and each choice you make to honor your body's wisdom.

You'll be able to use the practices you've discovered as life tools and companions as you continue to explore your inner landscape. Imagine a life in which somatic exercises are not just a routine but a way of life—one in which weight loss is just one of the many fruits of your efforts and well-being is the soil in which you deeply root yourself. This is the future of flourishing.

Growth and Gratitude We are grateful that you have included this book in your journey. May the somatic awareness seeds planted here bear fruit and grow into a garden of healthy movement and joy.

Step forward on the final page with the grace of a loved body, the strength of an empowered body, and the lightness of a freed body. May you always move with love, live with a purpose, and thrive in the radiant light of well-being as you dance with life.

www.ingramcontent.com/pod-product-compliance
Lightning Source LLC
Chambersburg PA
CBHW051854250726
48659CB00006B/2201